Basic guide to human trafficking for healthcare workers

By Anna May Xu

Table of contents

Chapter 1: Introduction 4
Definition 4
Smuggling and human trafficking 4
Force 6
Fraud 6
Coercion 6
Use of force 7
Types of trafficking 8

Chapter 2: Labor trafficking 10
Henry's Turkey Service 12
Signal Processing 16
Live-in nannies, cooks, and domestic servants 18

Chapter 3: Sex trafficking 20

Chapter 4: Identifying trafficking victims 22
River metaphor 23
Dual approaches to human trafficking 24
Risk factors for trafficking 26
Red flags 28
Barriers that prevent identification 32

Chapter 5: Interviewing victims of human trafficking 36

    Trauma 37
    Screening vs. universal education 40
    Screening tools 41
    Universal education tools 45
    Seeing patients alone 50
    Interpreters 52
Chapter 6: Reporting and treating trafficking victims 54
    Mandatory reporting 54
    The needs of a trafficking victim 56
    Preventing and treating human trafficking victims. 58
    Protective factors 61

Chapter 1: Introduction

Definition

Human trafficking is a crime that involves the exploitation of someone through the use of force, fraud, or coercion. This definition comes from the **Trafficking Victims Protection Act (TVPA) of 2000**.

Smuggling and human trafficking

People sometimes conflate human trafficking and smuggling.

Smugglers help people cross borders unlawfully. These people will often pay smugglers upfront for this service. The crime of smuggling ends at the border. Once the victims reach the border, the smugglers release them. Smuggling is a violation of a physical border and the autonomy of a government.

Human trafficking is forcing people to labor or engage in conduct for the benefit of the trafficker, without an endpoint. This is an abuse of the human rights of that individual. Trafficking also requires no movement. It can happen in private homes.

Trafficking Victims Protection Act (TVPA)

Actions for the purpose of

- commercial sexual exploitation
- forced labor

By the means of

- Force
- Coercion
- Fraud

*exception: minors who do commercial sex work are always human trafficking victims, regardless of force, fraud, or coercion

With action of

- recruiting
- harboring
- transporting
- providing
- obtaining

* in sex trafficking, there is also patronizing, soliciting, and advertising

Force

Force involves the use of serious physical harm or physical restraint. Physical violence such as beatings, rape, and physical confinement are common tactics to control victims, especially in the early stages of victimization.

Fraud

People can be lured into human trafficking by fraud, or false promises regarding employment, wages, working conditions, or other matters. For example, someone might travel to another country under the promise of well-paying work at a farm or factory but find themselves in forced labor. Sex trafficking victims are commonly lured by jobs that promise modeling or nanny work.

Coercion

Coercion involves the threat of serious harm or physical restraints. Traffickers will commonly threaten to report people to immigration, so they'll be deported or threaten to harm family members.

Use of force

Although traffickers do use normal sorts of force, like fences, chains, and locks, they often trap their victims with "**invisible chains**." Common examples of invisible chains are as threats, imposed debts, physical and emotional violence, drug addiction, display of weapons, and isolation. Industries that are underregulated and underpaid often use trafficked labor. This includes restaurant work, agricultural work, factories, nail salons, and domestic work.

Types of trafficking

US law divides human trafficking is divided into two categories: **labor trafficking** and **sex trafficking**. There is an important age distinction for sex trafficking – all people under age 18 who are exploited for commercial sex are considered to be trafficked.

Labor trafficking	Sex trafficking
Recruitment, harboring, transportation, provision, or obtaining of a person	Recruitment, harboring, transportation, provision, patronizing, or obtaining of a person
For labor or services Through force, fraud, or coercion	For a commercial sex act Through force, fraud, or coercion **or** person is under 18
For subjection to involuntary servitude, peonage, debt bondage, or slavery	

Chapter 2: Labor trafficking

Involuntary servitude relies on threats of violence, coercion and abuse of legal process, and fear tactics to force someone to continue working.

Debt bondage is manipulating debt to force someone to keep working. In American history, the most prominent example of this is the **company store scheme**. In the old railway and coal industry, workers were required to live far away and in a town that was owned by the company. Not only did the company set the wages for their workers, but they also set the prices for housing, food, uniforms, equipment, and other goods. Companies set the wages and prices in a way that the workers effectively made no money. They were trapped in that employment.

Involuntary servitude	Debt bondage or peonage
Threats of violence to victims or families	Forced to work off debt, may stem from agreement
Psychological coercion, including locked doors, guards, isolation	No choice in where or how to work off the debt
Abuse of legal process, including threats or deportation and debtors' prisons	Fees take all or nearly all the pay, so debt cannot be meaningfully reduced over time
	Example: company store scheme, in which a company coerces its employees to shop at its own store

Henry's Turkey Service

In 2013, the Equal Employment Opportunity Commission awarded $240 million to 32 intellectually disabled men who had been controlled for decades by a Texas-based poultry processing plant in Iowa. In the 1960s, Henry's Turkey Service, also known as Hill County Farms, started employing men who were released from Texas mental institutions. They were trafficked out of Texas and into Iowa, where they led isolated lives, away from their friends, family, and community.

Henry's Turkey Service paid these men $65 a month to remove innards from slaughtered turkeys. This came out to 41 cents an hour. The supervisors at Henry's forced the men to work long hours to keep the processing line moving and denied them backroom breaks.

Their supervisors also verbally and physically abused their workers. A common punishment for violating company policy was to be taken out to the garage and forced to walk around a pole, where they would either have to carry heavy objects or get hit and kicked. One man had been kicked in the groin so often that his testicles were swollen.

The company docked the men's wages and Social Security disability benefits, while claiming it was to pay for the cost of their care and lodging. However, Henry's deliberately chose to not provide the men with medical care. The men suffered from diabetes, hypertension, malnutrition, festering fungal infections. One man had hands that were infected from constant contact with turkey blood. Severe dental problems went untreated. One man couldn't chew a waffle due to the poor state of his teeth.

The workers were housed in a 100-year-old bunkhouse in Atalissa, Iowa and bussed in daily to work. Their house was infested with rodents, bugs, and cockroaches. The windows were boarded up, so there was little ventilation or light. The windows were broken, so when it rained, their beds got wet. The roof was leaky and covered with mildew, grease, and mice droppings. The men were locked in their bedrooms at night. One man was even handcuffed to his bed. The house was full of fire hazards. A fire marshal immediately condemned the building and said that it was the worst he had seen in nearly 3,000 inspections.

Company president Kenneth Henry, 72, testified that over 45 years, Henry's Turkey Service sent 1,500 mentally disabled men to labor camps in seven states. Henry's Turkey Service didn't have enough assets to cover the $240 million award and went bankrupt.

US · Published May 1, 2013 · Last Update November 21, 2015

Jury awards $240 million to 32 mentally disabled Iowa turkey plant workers for years of abuse

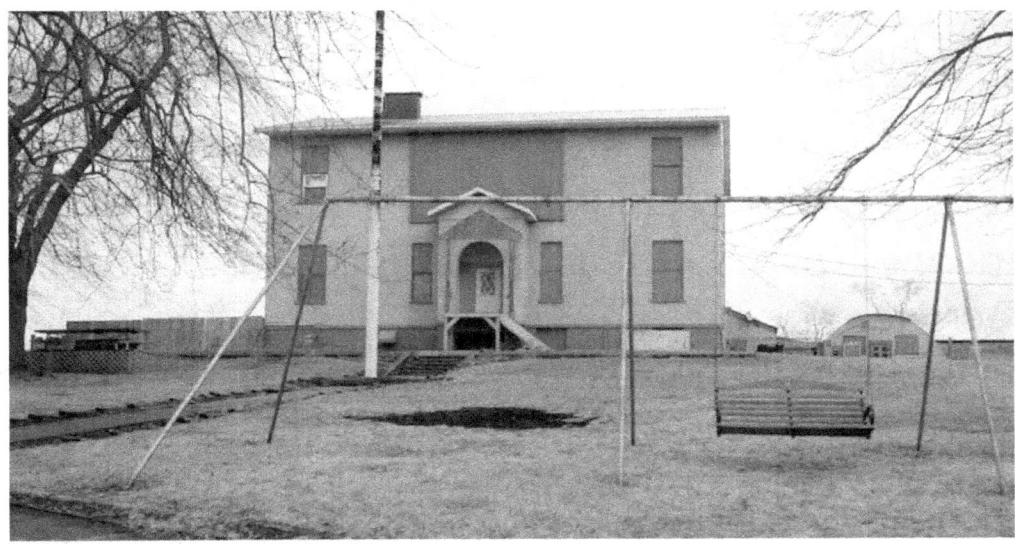

IOWA CITY, Iowa – For decades, the lives of 32 mentally disabled Iowa turkey processing plant workers were controlled by their Texas-based employer, which profited handsomely by hiring them out.

Regardless of sickness or injury, they were driven from the dilapidated, bug-infested bunkhouse where they were housed to their 41-cents-an-hour jobs removing the slaughtered birds' innards. Day and night, at work and at home, their overseers subjected them to verbal and physical abuse that left them with "broken hearts, broken spirits, shattered dreams, and ultimately broken lives," a government attorney said.

On Wednesday, they made history when a federal jury in Davenport awarded them $240 million — the largest verdict in the 48-year history of the Equal Employment Opportunity Commission, which sued on their behalf.

It's unlikely the men's former employer, the now-defunct Henry's Turkey Service, of Goldthwaite, Texas, has anywhere near enough remaining assets to cover the $7.5 million in damages each man was awarded. But federal officials vowed to recover every last cent they could for the men, who had been "virtually enslaved" for many years, according to developmental psychologist Sue Gant, who interviewed them at length for the EEOC.

"That discrimination caused them such irreparable harm, and the jury got that. They

Signal Processing

In 2015, a New Orleans jury awarded $14 million to five Indian men who had been trafficked to the United States and forced to work under debt bondage. Over 200 workers sued Signal Processing in one of the largest labor trafficking cases in U.S. history.

In 2005, Signal Processing recruited about 500 Indian men to repair the oil rigs that were damaged by Hurricane Katrina. The workers paid $10,000 upfront to recruiters for the employment visas, after being falsely promised permanent residency in the United States. After the men arrived, Signal charged the men $1,050 per month to live in guarded labor camps. Up to 24 men could live in an 1,800-square-foot, squalid, dirty trailer.

Signal Processing also charged their workers for housing, food, supplies, and tools and deducted these fees from their paychecks.

Signal Processing saved more than $8 million by hiring the Indian workers. After the trial, Signal International of Mobile, Alabama, filed for Chapter 11 bankruptcy protection.

Indian workers awarded millions after US firm found guilty of trafficking

Five men awarded $14m after being lured to US to help repair damage after Hurricane Katrina

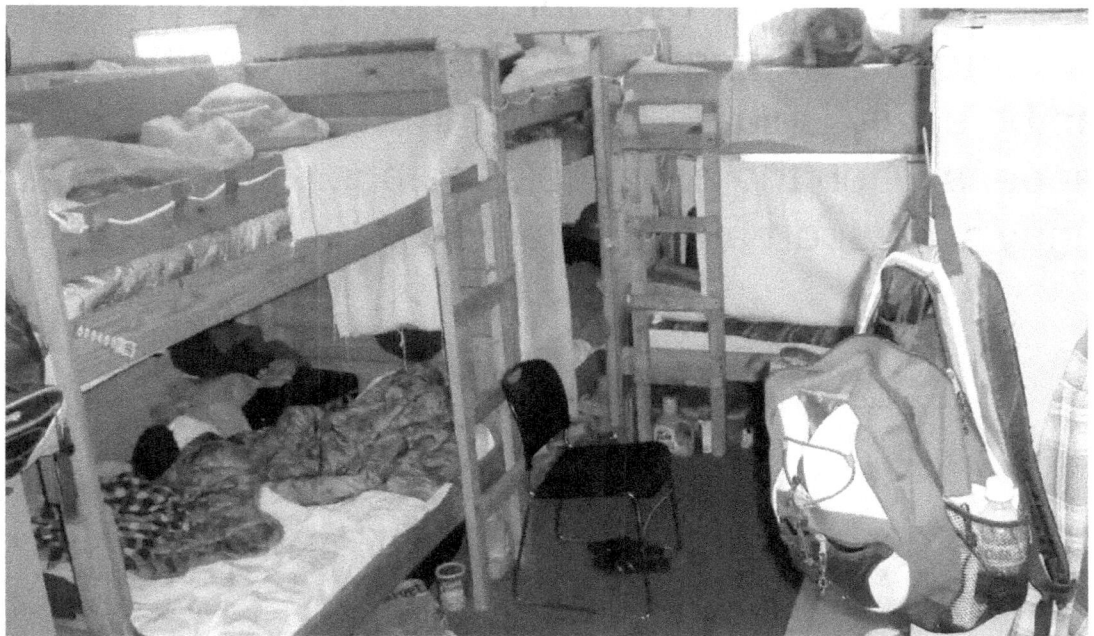

▲ Inside a work camp used by Indian workers in the Signal shipyards in Pascagoula, Mississippi. A New Orleans jury awarded $14 million to five Indian men who were lured to the United States and forced to work under inhumane conditions after Hurricane Katrina. Photograph: Handout/Reuters

Reuters

Thu 19 Feb 2015 00.07 EST

A New Orleans jury on Wednesday awarded $14m to five Indian men who were lured to the United States and forced to work under inhumane conditions after Hurricane Katrina by a ship repair firm and its codefendants.

After a four-week trial, the US District Court jury ruled that Alabama-based Signal International was guilty of labour trafficking, fraud, racketeering and discrimination and ordered it to pay $12m. Its co-defendants, a New Orleans lawyer and an India-based recruiter, were also found guilty and ordered to pay an additional $915,000 each.

Live-in nannies, cooks, and domestic servants

Trafficking doesn't require movement. Someone can be trafficked in their own home. People who provide childcare or healthcare in someone's private home can be easily isolated. Usually, this sort of trafficking happens when the household members take away the nanny's passport and isolate her.

Chapter 3: Sex trafficking

Sex trafficking is the recruitment, harboring, transportation, provision, obtaining, patronizing, or soliciting of someone for the purposes of a commercial sex act. If the person is over 18, then the commercial sex act has to involve force, fraud, or coercion. If the person is under 18, then no force, fraud, or coercion is required.

A **commercial sex act** is any sex in which something of value is given to or received by any person. Common trades are cash, drugs, a place to stay, a cell phone, and food. Sex acts also include soliciting and patronizing someone for the purpose of a commercial sex act.

Here is a graph from the Polaris Project that details the number and types of human trafficking cases in the United States.

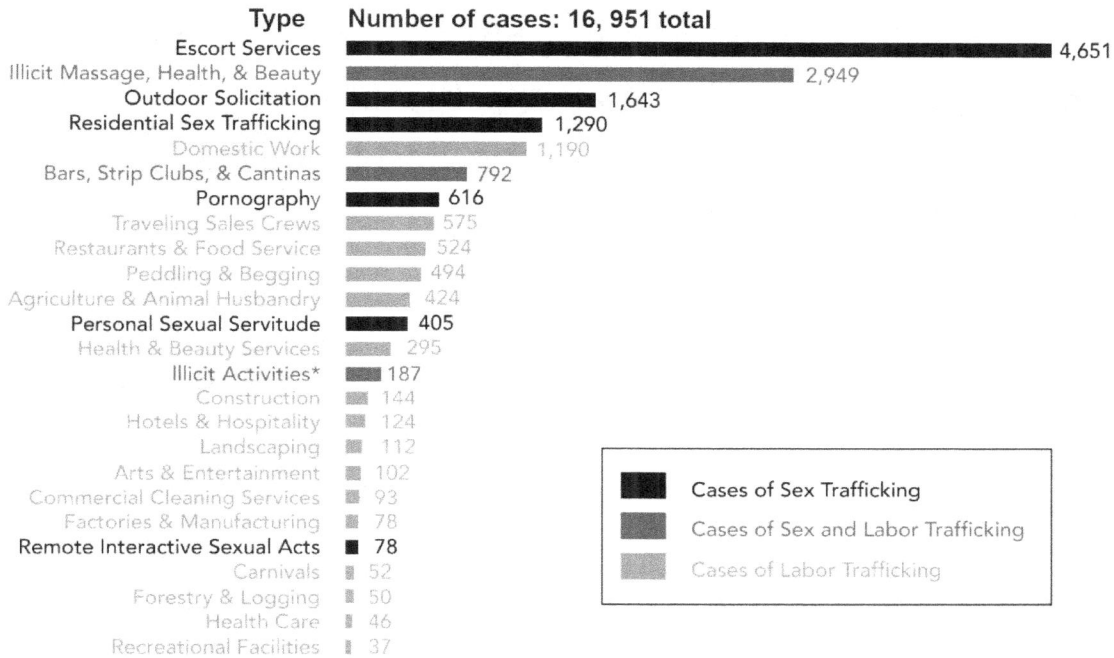

https://polarisproject.org/resources/the-typology-of-modern-slavery-defining-sex-and-labor-trafficking-in-the-united-states/

Chapter 4: Identifying trafficking victims

68% of trafficking victims sought healthcare while they were being trafficked. However, healthcare practitioners didn't always recognize that their patients were trafficking victims.

Health Care and Human Trafficking: We are Seeing the Unseen

Makini Chisolm-Straker, Susie Baldwin, Bertille Gaïgbé-Togbé, Nneka Ndukwe, Pauline N Johnson, Lynne D Richardson

Abstract

Objectives: This study aimed to build the evidence base around human trafficking (HT) and health in the U.S. by employing a quantitative approach to exploring the notion that health care providers encounter this population. Furthermore, this study sought to describe the health care settings most frequented by victims of human trafficking.

Methods: This was an anonymous, retrospective study of survivors of U.S.-based human trafficking.

Results: One hundred and seventy-three participants who endured U.S.-based human trafficking were surveyed. The majority (68%, n=117) of participants were seen by a health care provider while being trafficked. Respondents most frequently reported visiting emergency/urgent care practitioners (56%), followed by primary care providers, dentists, and obstetricians/gynecologists (OB/GYNs).

Conclusions: While health care providers are serving this patient population, they do not consistently identify them as victims of human trafficking.

https://pubmed.ncbi.nlm.nih.gov/27524764/

River metaphor

The river metaphor is in vogue as a way to address root causes in public health issues. You're sitting on the banks of a river when you notice that someone is floating by. He's drowning so you go in and save him. As soon as he's safe, you notice another person floating by. He's also drowning, and you save him too. Then you see another person drowning, and so on. Eventually, as you're lying on the bank, exhausted from saving so many people, you wonder why there are so many drownings. You walk upstream to see why so many so many people are falling into the river. It turns out that there's a cliff that gives a great view of the river. It looks deceptively safe, but once people get on the cliff, they fall down and into the river.

At this point, the public health people will talk about upstream and downstream activities. Downstream activities are hiring lifeguards at the river, buying better floatation devices, putting up warning signs that the river is dangerous, and arresting people for drowning. Upstream activities are finding out why people are falling into the river, putting up fences around the cliff, and getting the local news to cover why the cliff is dangerous.

Dual approaches to human trafficking

The **criminal justice system** helps people who are already drowning downstream. The criminal response punishes traffickers and recovers victims. The services that it provides are short-term and focus on preparing victims to be witnesses against their traffickers in court.

The **public health system** is part of the upstream safety system. They prevent people prevent from falling into the river in the first place. The public health response addresses the underlying causes so they can prevent harm from occurring in the first place. Although the entry level policies are raising awareness and basic education, public health aims to find the root causes of trafficking and then change the conditions that cause it.

Upstream

Public health framework

purpose: prevent and treat harm to patients and clients

- long-term process
- focus on individual and population-level health
- community-based
- support of individual, family, and community

Downstream

Criminal justice framework

purpose: punish traffickers and recover victims

- defined timeframe
- justice-oriented
- based on government
- upholds legal framework

Risk factors for trafficking

Individuals with the following characteristics are at a higher risk of being trafficked:

- History of abuse or neglect
- Social disconnection, stigma, or disconnection
- Homeless, runaway, or "thrown away"
- Exclusion

These populations are disproportionately affected by trafficking:

- Refugees
- Migrant and seasonal workers, with H-2A and H-2B visas
- Youths who were "systems-involved," such as juvenile justice or foster care
- Disconnected youth, unaccompanied minors, runaway youths, and homeless youths
- Native Americans
- Lesbian, gay, bisexual, and transexuals
- People with physical or cognitive disabilities
- Survivors of violence or other crimes

Red flags

Here are some signs that someone is being trafficked.

Missing paperwork
- Lack of personal documents
- Lack of travel documents

Sexual and drug-related injuries
- High number of sexual partners
- Multiple pregnancies or terminations
- Frequent treatment for sexually transmitted infections
- Communicable and non-communicable diseases, such as tuberculosis or hepatitis
- Substance use
- Dental issues

Physical injuries

- Bruising and burns
- Untreated or undertreated workplace injuries
- Physical impacts of long-term trauma
- Tattoos, burns, or scarring that indicates branding

Lung injuries

- Respiratory issues
- Exposure to toxic chemicals

Behavioral red flags

- Unawareness of age, location, and time
- Inability to focus or concentrate
- Confusing or contradicting stories
- Reserved, avoids interaction, or provides limited information
- Protects the person who hurt them
- Minimizes abuse

Psychological red flags

- Depression and anxiety disorders
- Psychological trauma

Sexual behavior

- Sexual acting out in children and young adolescents
- Knowledge about sex outside of typical range for age

School environment

- Changes in behavior, no longer coming to school when they should, wearing the wrong clothing based on the season

Work environment

- Unsafe working conditions
- No pay or low pay
- Sexual harassment
- Not allowed to take adequate breaks, eat, or drink
- Recruited for different work than currently doing
- Working to pay off a debt
- Threats of deportation

Housing

- Unsafe living conditions
- Living at work or living in overcrowded locations
- Living at a motel
- Living with non-family members who are several years older
- Homeless minors

Handlers

- Constantly accompanied by a person who won't leave them alone
- Accompanied by another person who answers for them and prevents them from speaking freely

Barriers that prevent identification

People who are being trafficked may hinder their own identification.

An individual's knowledge barriers

- Limited literacy and education that hinders their ability to communicate
- Language barrier
- Lack of understanding of legal rights
- Lack of identification and other paper records
- Lack of awareness of victimization

An individual's fears

- Fear that someone reporting them could lead to being returned to an abusive home, foster care, or jail
- Fear of law enforcement and deportation
- Fear that traffickers will cause harm to themselves or family members

An individual's psychological barriers

- Feels hopelessness, helplessness, shame, or guilt
- Feels complicit in an illegal act
- Trauma bonding with trafficker or other victims
- Distrusts healthcare provides or authority figures

Healthcare workers can also fail to identify trafficking victims.

Lack of training for providers
- Inadequate knowledge about human trafficking
- Inadequate knowledge of federal and state human trafficking laws
- Fears violating Health Insurance Portability and Accountability (HIPAA) rules
- Inadequate trauma-informed care training
- Misidentifies the case

Lack of access to services for providers
- Lack of access to translators and interpreters
- Lacks good referral options

Incorrect preconceptions about human trafficking

- Has preconceived notions of what human trafficking victims look like or how they behave
- Attributes behaviors to cultural stereotypes
- Presence of bias or victim-blaming attitudes
- "Checks off boxes" without seeing the full situation
- Doesn't believe it's their role to get involved
- Believes it'll be too time-consuming or complex
- Believes that the trafficked individual is hostile, unresponsive, or telling a rehearsed story

Chapter 5: Interviewing victims of human trafficking

For healthcare workers, the goal of interviewing trafficking victims isn't disclosure of the trafficking itself – it's to ensure their safety, well-being, and provide services and resources. The first thing to keep in mind is that violence affects people's development and ability to cope. It's important to be sensitive to their trauma and avoid re-traumatizing them.

Trauma

Trauma results from emotionally or physically harmful events or circumstances. This harm has lasting effects and negatively affects people's mental, physical, social, emotional, or spiritual well-being, especially if the traumatic events happened during childhood. Risky behaviors such as substance use and mental health conditions have been linked with traumatic experienced.

Childhood trauma

A trafficking victim's first trauma usually isn't the trafficking event itself. Adverse childhood events (ACEs) are stressful or traumatic events that happens during a person's formative years. They have long-term effects on a person's health and lifespan. Common ACEs are abuse, neglect, and household dysfunction.

Secondary trauma

Secondary trauma results from helping or wanting to help someone who has experienced trauma. If staff experience secondary trauma, not only can their job performance deteriorate, but they may also become personally affected. These negative effects are exacerbated if the workplace has an unsupportive or toxic environment.

The **emotional** effects of secondary trauma include:

- Anger
- Fear
- Shame
- Physical illness
- Emotional exhaustion
- Grief or despair
- Sensitivity to violence
- Cynicism or seriousness

The **physical** side effects of secondary trauma are:

- Illness
- Intrusive thoughts
- Absenteeism and turnover

Journal of Public Child Welfare
Volume 9, 2015 - Issue 2

Relationship Between Vicarious Traumatization and Turnover Among Child Welfare Professionals

Jennifer Sean Middleton & Cathryn C. Potter

Pages 195-216 | Received 27 Jul 2014, Accepted 18 Feb 2015, Published online: 18 May 2015

Abstract

Child welfare professionals work on the front lines with maltreated children and their families every day. The very nature of the work can have a significant impact on their emotional well being and ability to effectively perform their jobs, potentially limiting quality service delivery and contributing to overall workforce capacity issues such a turnover. This study examined the relationship between vicarious traumatization and turnover among 1,192 child welfare professionals in five different child welfare organizations across four states. Propositions from constructivist self-development theory (CSDT) were utilized to examine the causal relationship between vicarious traumatization and child welfare professionals' intent to leave their organization. Structural Equation Modeling (SEM) was used to assess the degree of fit between the observed data and a hypothesized theoretical model examining the relationship between vicarious trauma and intent to leave. Findings from SEM analyses revealed a significant relationship between vicarious traumatization and intent to leave. This finding indicates that child welfare professionals who experienced higher rates of vicarious traumatization are more likely to leave their organization. Implications of these findings for theory, practice, and research are delineated.

Keywords: workforce issues, organizations/systems, vicarious traumatization, turnover, structural equation modeling

Screening vs. universal education

There are two schools of thought on identifying victims of trafficking.

The first one is **screening**, which is used when red flags indicate that a patient is a human trafficking victim. A screening questionnaire asks patients a standardized set of yes-no questions about human trafficking. These questionnaires identify whether the patient is involved in human trafficking and which services they need. The provider or the insurance then determines which services that the patient qualifies for. This method is better for healthcare providers who see patients on a short-term basis, such as an emergency department.

The second one is **universal education**, which is when the provider inquiries about the patient's needs while simultaneously educating them about how interpersonal relationships, socioeconomic, and environmental factors affect their situation. Then the patient and the provider work together to determine which services are appropriate for that patient. This method is better for providers who see patients on a long-term basis, such as behavioral health clinics.

Screening tools

There are several screening tools available.

Human Trafficking Screening Tool (HTST)

This tool identifies minors who have been trafficked.

Human Trafficking Screening Tool Questions

#	Did someone you work for...	Hypothesized domain
1	Physically force you to do something you didn't feel comfortable doing	Force
2	Lock you up, restrain you, or prevent you from leaving	Force
3	Physically harm you in any way (beat, slap, hit, kick, punch, burn)	Force
4	Trick you into doing different work than was promised	Fraud
5	Make you sign a document without understanding what it stated, like a work contract	Fraud
6	Refuse to pay you or pay less than they promised	Fraud
7	Restrict or control where you went or who you talked to	Coercion
8	Deprive you of sleep, food, water, or medical care	Coercion
9	Not let you contact family or friends, even when you weren't working	Coercion
10	Keep all or most of your money or pay	Coercion
11	Keep your ID documents (e.g., ID card, license, passport, social security card, birth certificate) from you	Coercion
12	Threaten to get you deported	Coercion
13	Threaten to harm you or your family or pet	Coercion
14	Physically harm or threaten a coworker or friend	Coercion
15	Force you to do something sexually that you didn't feel comfortable doing	Commercial sex exploitation
16	Put your photo on the Internet to find clients to trade sex with	Commercial sex exploitation
17	Force you to engage in sexual acts with family, friends, or business associates for money or favors	Commercial sex exploitation
18	Encourage or pressure you to do sexual acts or have sex, including taking sexual photos or videos	Commercial sex exploitation
19	Force you to trade sex for money, shelter, food, or anything else through online websites, escort services, street prostitution, informal arrangements, brothels, fake massage businesses, or strip clubs	Commercial sex exploitation

https://www.urban.org/research/publication/pretesting-human-trafficking-screening-tool-child-welfare-and-runaway-and-homeless-youth-systems/view/full_report

Toolkit and Guide: Adult Human Trafficking Screening

This tool identifies adults who have been trafficked. It's supposed to be used in conjunction with the Human Trafficking Screening Tool.

https://nhttac.acf.hhs.gov/resources/toolkit-adult-human-trafficking-screening-tool-and-guide

Question	Respondent Answers
1. Sometimes lies are used to trick people into accepting a job that doesn't exist, and they get trapped in a job or situation they never wanted. Have you ever experienced this, or are you in a situation where you think this could happen?	Yes No Declined to Answer Don't Know
2. Sometimes people make efforts to repay a person who provided them with transportation, a place to stay, money, or something else they needed. The person they owe money to may require them to do things if they have difficulty paying because of the debt. Have you ever experienced this, or are you in a situation where you think this could happen?	Yes No Declined to Answer Don't Know
3. Sometimes people do unfair, unsafe, or even dangerous work or stay in dangerous situation because if they don't, someone might hurt them or someone they love. Have you ever experienced this, or are you in a situation where you think this could happen?	Yes No Declined to Answer Don't Know
4. Sometimes people are not allowed to keep or hold on to their own identification or travel documents. Have you ever experienced this, or are you in a situation where you think this could happen?	Yes No Declined to Answer Don't Know
5. Sometimes people work for someone or spend time with someone who does not let them contact their family, spend time with their friends, or go where they want when they want. Have you ever experienced this, or are you in a situation where you think this could happen?	Yes No Declined to Answer Don't Know
6. Sometimes people live where they work or where the person in charge tells them to live, and they're not allowed to live elsewhere. Have you ever experienced this, or are you in a situation where you think this could happen?	Yes No Declined to Answer Don't Know
7. Sometimes people are told to lie about their situation, including the kind of work they do. Has anyone ever told you to lie about the kind of work you're doing or will be doing?	Yes No Declined to Answer Don't Know
8. Sometimes people are hurt or threatened, or threats are made to their family or loved ones, or they are forced to do things they do not want to do in order to make money for someone else or to pay off a debt to them. Have you ever experienced this, or are you in a situation where you think this could happen?	Yes No Declined to Answer Don't Know

Quick Youth Indicators for Trafficking (QYIT)

This tool identifies homeless and runaway youth, age 18-22, who have been trafficked.

Quick Youth Indicators of Trafficking (QYIT)

1. It is not uncommon for young people to stay in work situations that are risky or even dangerous, simply because they have no other options. Have you ever worked, or done other things, in a place that made you feel scared or unsafe?

2. Sometimes people are prevented from leaving an unfair or unsafe work situation by their employers. Have you ever been afraid to leave or quit a work situation due to fears of violence or threats of harm to yourself or your family?

3. Sometimes young people who are homeless or who have difficulties with their families have very few options to survive or fulfill their basic needs, such as food and shelter. Have you ever received anything in exchange for sex (e.g.: a place to stay, gifts, or food)?

4. Sometimes employers don't want people to know about the kind of work they have young employees doing. To protect themselves, they ask their employees to lie about the kind of work they are involved in. Have you ever worked for someone who asked you to lie while speaking to others about the work you do?

https://www.sciencedirect.com/science/article/pii/S0190740918307540

Universal education tools

Here are two universal education tools for identifying victims of human trafficking.

PEARR

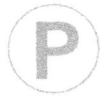
Provide Privacy

1. Discuss sensitive topics **alone** and in **safe, private setting** (ideally private room with closed doors). If companion refuses to be separated, then this may be an indicator of abuse, neglect, or violence.** Strategies to speak with patient alone: State requirement for private exam or need for patient to be seen alone for radiology, urine test, etc.

   Note: Companions are not appropriate interpreters, regardless of communication abilities. If patient indicates preference to use

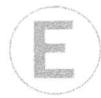
Educate

2. Educate patient in manner that is **nonjudgmental** and **normalizes** sharing of information. Example: "I educate all of my patients about [fill in the blank] because violence is so common in our society, and violence has a big impact on our health, safety, and well-being." **Use a brochure or safety card** to review information about abuse, neglect, or violence, and

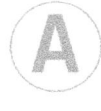
Ask

3. Allow time for discussion with patient. Example: "Is there anything you'd like to share with me? Do you feel like anyone is hurting your health, safety, or well-being?"** If available and when appropriate, use **evidence-based tools** to screen patient for abuse, neglect, or violence.**

   Note: All women of reproductive age should be intermittently screened for intimate partner violence (USPSTF Grade B).

4. If there are indicators of victimization, **ASK** about concerns. Example: "I've noticed [insert risk factor/indicator] and I'm concerned for your

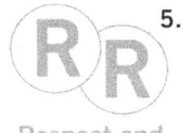
Respect and Respond

5. If patient denies victimization or declines assistance, then **respect patient's wishes.** If you have **concerns about patient's safety,** offer hotline card or other information about resources that can assist in event of emergency (e.g., local shelter, crisis hotline).** Otherwise, if patient accepts/requests assistance with accessing services, then **provide personal introduction**

CUES

The CUES tool requires healthcare providers to start conversations about human trafficking by giving their patient two safety cards or mini brochures.

C: Confidentiality

Every visit has to have a portion in which the provider sees the patient alone. The provider has to say that they bring up the topic of relationship violence and human trafficking with every patient. You should know your state's mandatory reporting laws and limits of confidentiality.

UE: Universal Education + Empowerment

Everyone gets information about how to prevent relationship violence, not just those who choose to disclose. One card is for the victim and the other is for a trusted family member or friend.

S: Support

After a patient discloses relationship violence or human trafficking, the provider should support the patient by warmly creating a care plan and referring them to other services.

How to ask questions

Sometimes how you ask a question is just as important as what the question actually is.

Asking questions when their handler or partner is sitting right next to them: If you ask, "is anyone hurting you at home?" when the abuser is right next to the victim, then it is unlikely you'll get a truthful answer.

Asking questions when you're typing at the computer or your back is turned: The patient may feel discouraged from being honest.

"I'm sorry to ask you these questions. It's a requirement of the clinic.": This may make the patient feel as if their situation isn't valid.

"Have you ever been hit, kicked, slapped, or choked by a partner at home?": These sorts of questions have a low disclosure rate.

Alternatives

Here are a few better ways to ask trafficking victims questions.

Make eye contact throughout the session: This makes the patient feel like their provider is taking them seriously.

Open with a framing statement such as, "We're started talking to all patients about safe relationships because it can impact your health.": This creates the context of the screening process.

Discuss confidentiality and the limits to confidentiality: Sometimes trafficking victims may have preconceptions on what healthcare providers will tell law enforcement officers. Healthcare providers should give a plain language brochure about confidentiality to their patients.

Ask, "Has your partner ever made you feel frightened or threatened in any way?": After asking this question, you should pay attention to both verbal and non-verbal responses.

Seeing patients alone

It's important to set a policy that encourages healthcare providers to see their patients alone for at least part of their visit, especially when the provider is conducting assessments and interventions.

Administrators can implement this culture change by orienting staff to the policy change and getting their buy-in. Afterwards, they should post the new policy in common areas, such as waiting rooms, exam rooms, and bathrooms.

New clinic policy

For patient privacy, every individual will be seen alone for some part of their visit. Thank you for your cooperation.

When you can't see every individual alone

Sometimes the patient's handler is hostile when asked to leave the patient. A clinic should have policies on:

- when to separate suspected trafficked from his victim
- what reason to give to the trafficked
- who will separate the two people
- what safety measures are need

Interpreters

Skilled and qualified interpreters are essential for communicating with patients who have limited English proficiency or speak a different language. Even when providers have an interpreter, they should use the same basic communication standards and etiquette that they would use when speaking directly to a patient

Interpreters should receive training so that they know:

- patient confidentiality and the limits of that confidentiality
- how to monitor people for signs of stress and then slow down or pause interviews, so the patient doesn't get overwhelmed
- to translate verbatim, even slang or swear words
- proper terminology so they don't unintentionally use words that are perceived as victim blaming
- to be prepared for secondary trauma, or being triggered or traumatized by the nature of the conversation

Clinic policies

The clinic should create the following policies for interpreters:

- How to determine when an interpreter is needed
- Who is the designated interviewer
- How to contact them
- What approach or interview style to use
- How to train interviewers

Chapter 6: Reporting and treating trafficking victims

After identifying trafficking victims and interviewing them, healthcare providers have to treat their patients, refer them to secondary services, and report them as mandated by state and federal law.

Mandatory reporting

Many states have laws that require healthcare providers to report people who they believe are being trafficked. Healthcare organizations have a responsibility to have policies in place and train their staff to do this in a way that won't traumatize their patients.

Required reporting laws vary state by state, so each healthcare organization will have to check up on what data they can and cannot share.

Federal laws

The **Trafficking Victims Protection Act (TVPA)** requires federal, state, and local officials to notify Health and Human Services within 24 hours of discovering a child who may be a foreign victim of trafficking.

The **Preventing Sex Trafficking and Strengthening Families Act** requires state child welfare agencies to report any missing children to law enforcement and the National Center for Missing and Exploited Children (NCMEC) within 24 hours.

Confidentiality and limits to confidentiality

As a note, Health Insurance Portability and Accountability Act (HIPAA) isn't designed to prevent trauma or crimes. Many trafficking situations don't fall under mandatory reporting. Healthcare providers and the victim can often decide which details they want to disclose to law enforcement officers.

The needs of a trafficking victim

A healthcare provider's ultimate goal for trafficking victims is to get them the help they need, both in the short-term and long-term.

General needs

Victims of human trafficking have the same basic needs as everyone else.

- Food
- Clothing
- Housing
- Transportation

Emergency needs

After a provider determines that their patient is a trafficking victim, the next step is to provide for the victim's immediate needs.

- Safety
- Shelter
- Medical care
- Intensive case management
- Treatment for substance use
- Dental care

Short-term needs

After their condition is stabilized, the victim will need these services

- Ongoing medical care, especially services for mental health and substance use
- Transportation to medical appointments
- Translation and interpretation services
- Legal assistance
- Access to secondary and referral services

Long-term needs

Lastly, the patient will need these services to integrate back into society and recover.

- Victim advocacy
- Legal services, especially for legal status and documentation
- Education
- English as a second language (ESL) classes
- Job training and placement
- Family reunification
- Parenting classes
- Spiritual or religious support

Preventing and treating human trafficking victims

Here's how healthcare providers can help victims of human trafficking.

	Patient **is not** being trafficked	Patient **is** being trafficked
Health harm is **absent** in patient	**Primary prevention:** Raising awareness in communities, school, or media	**Secondary prevention:** Identification and screening of potential victims in clinics or schools
Health harm is **present** in patient	**Long-term care:** Long-term care and behavioral treatment to survivors	**Tertiary prevention:** Acute visit to emergency department

Table adapted from Kimberly Chang and A. Seiji Hayashi's The Role of Community Health Centers in Addressing Human Trafficking

Primary prevention

Primary prevention helps people who have not experienced trafficking, injuries, or traumas. The usual method for primary prevention is education. In this case, it would be education about safe relationships, labor and sexual exploitation, and reproductive health issues. Organizations can raise awareness about such issues in the community, media, or schools.

Secondary prevention

Secondary prevention helps patients who are being trafficked but have no yet experienced health harm. For example, a person could be in the grooming stage of being trafficked by someone she is in love with but has not yet been beaten by the trafficked or experienced a sexually transmitted infection. The most common secondary prevention interventions are screening tools and training staff to use those tools.

Tertiary prevention

Tertiary prevention helps patients who are currently being trafficked and are experiencing health issues. This is the classic case of a trafficking victim who gets treated in the emergency room.

Long-term care

Long-term care is for people who are no longer being trafficked or no longer meet the criteria for being trafficked, and now need healthcare for their long-term needs. For example, a person who had been trafficked in the past and had transitioned out of labor exploitation may still have coronary artery disease, human immunodeficiency virus, post-traumatic stress disorder, depression, anxiety, or children with their trafficker. Another common example is a child who had been sex trafficked, but once they turn 18 years old, may not be able to prove force, fraud, or coercion and thus no longer meets the criteria for being a victim of sex trafficking.

Protective factors

Public health workers, such as social workers and behavioral health specialists, work with community health organizations to prevent both labor and sex trafficking. A popular phrase is "you cannot arrest your way out of trafficking" – meaning you have to address both population-level and individual-level factors that prevent trafficking in the first place.

- Stable housing and household income
- Positive role models and mentors
- Community engagement
- Increased awareness of trafficking
- Skill development and vocational training
- Substance use treatment

www.ingramcontent.com/pod-product-compliance
Lightning Source LLC
Chambersburg PA
CBHW080903220526
45466CB00011BA/3452